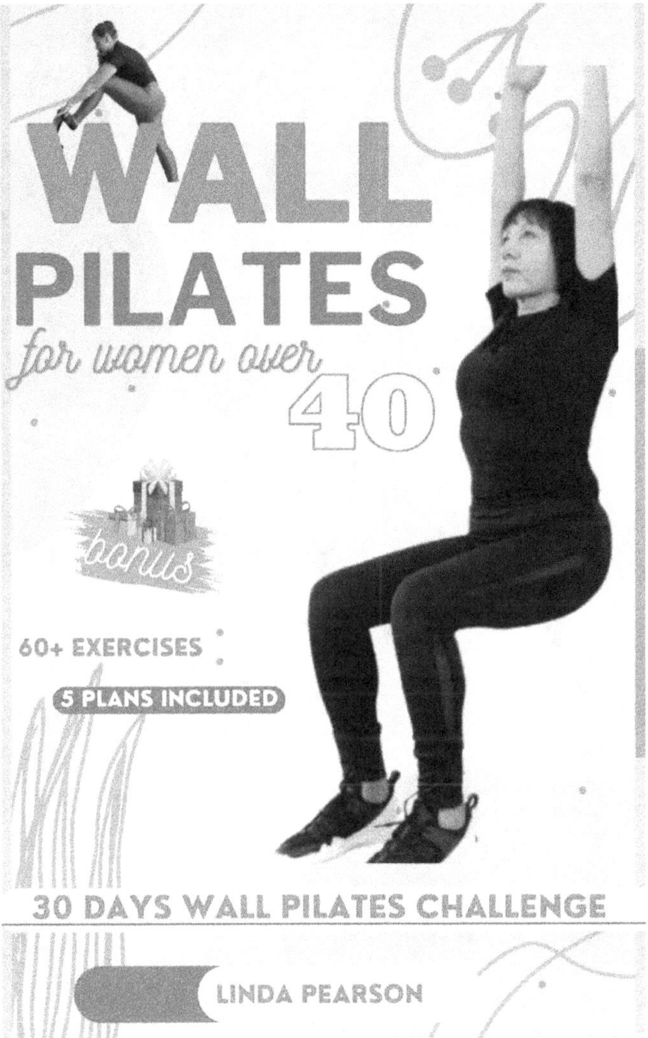

WALL PILATES

for women over 40

40

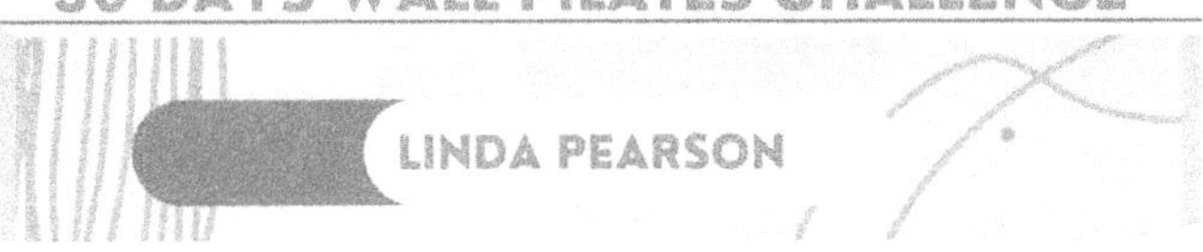

bonus

60+ EXERCISES

5 PLANS INCLUDED

30 DAYS WALL PILATES CHALLENGE

LINDA PEARSON

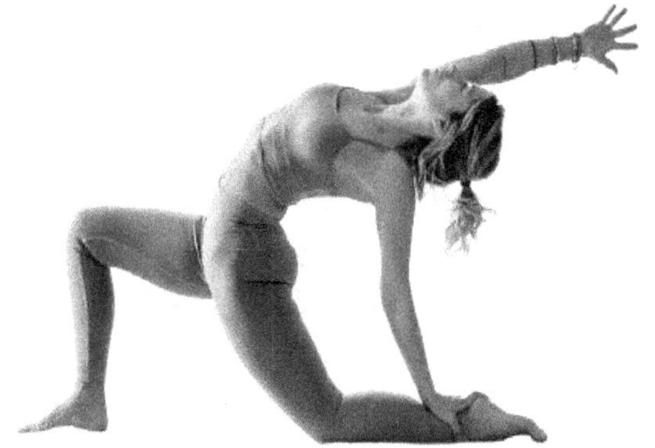

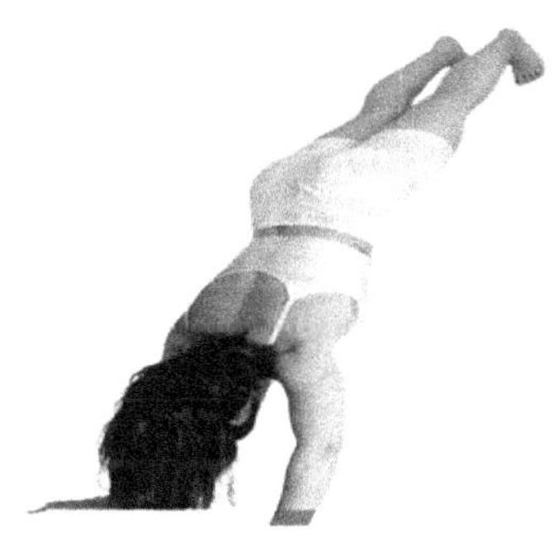

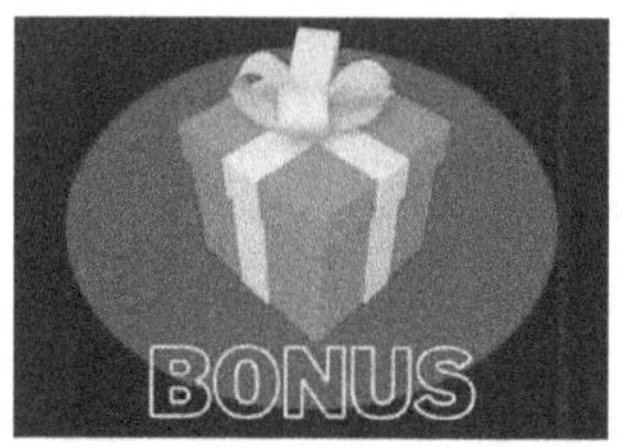

SCAN THE QR CODE TO GET YOUR FREE HOME MADE GREEN SMOOTHIE RECIPE BOOK

YOUR EXERCISE LOG AND 4-WEEKS WORKOUT PLAN JOURNAL AWAITS YOU AT THE END OF THE BOOK.

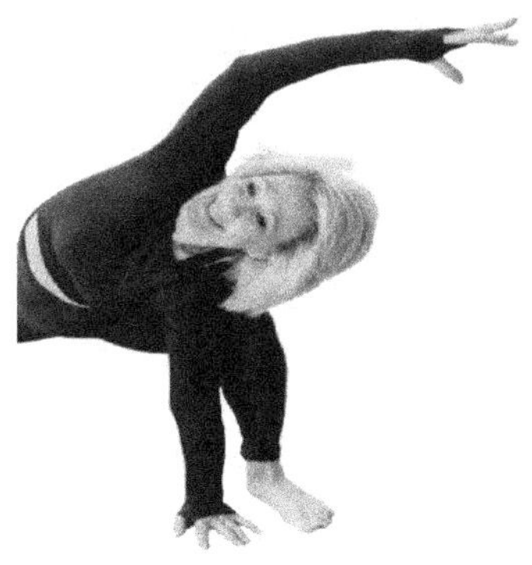

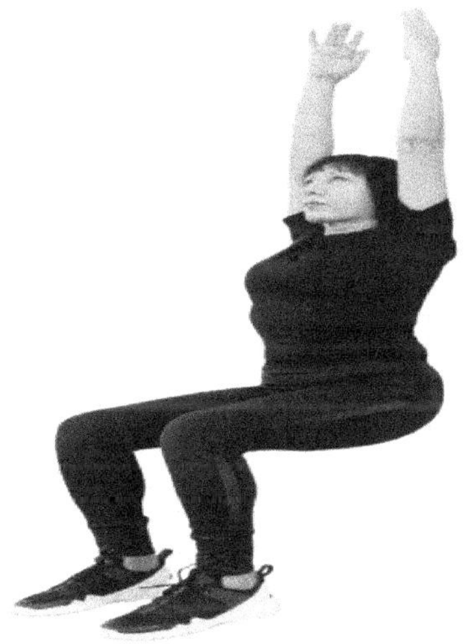

Table of contents

Introduction

Every person eventually searches for a place where their mind, body, and soul can come together in perfect harmony inside the maze of life. This haven can be found in the world of Pilates, a transforming training style that has stood the test of time, for many women over the age of 40. However, there are many different methods and techniques throughout the wide Pilates universe. In this investigation, we'll delve into the world of Pilates, looking at its many variations before shining a light on Wall Pilates and why it works so well for women over 40.

Pilates variations

Joseph Pilates invented Pilates in the early 20th century, and since then it has developed into a comprehensive discipline that is appropriate for people of various ages and fitness levels. The most common ones are enumerated below:

Pilates exercises are performed on a padded mat and emphasize balance, flexibility, and core strength. It's a terrific place to start for novices and may be modified for people of different fitness levels.

Pilates using a Reformer:

The Reformer is a specialized piece of equipment that uses springs and pulleys to create resistance during Pilates exercises. It works wonders for strengthening muscles and enhancing posture.

Aerial Pilates:

This variation of Pilates literally raises the bar by having participants carry out their movements while suspended in a silk hammock. Your core will be tested as you strengthen your upper body with aerial Pilates.

Clinical Pilates

Physical therapists frequently suggest Clinical Pilates since it is designed to address certain injuries or ailments. It is a rehabilitation strategy that encourages recovery and healing.

Contemporary Pilates:

This adaptation of Pilates uses equipment like stability balls, resistance bands, and magic circles to increase the intensity and variety of the workout.

Wall exercises: Let's focus now on Wall Pilates, the main actor in our production.

The Value of Wall Pilates for Senior Women

Women over 40 should give the lesser-known but highly effective form of wall Pilates a special place in their exercise regimen. This is why:

1. **Improved Support and Stability**: Maintaining balance and stability becomes more important as we age. Wall Pilates makes use of a wall's support to provide a safe environment for exercises. This is especially helpful for women who might worry about injuries brought on by poor balance.

2. Easy on the Joints: Traditional Pilates exercises can occasionally be difficult on the joints, particularly for people who already have joint problems from aging. With its emphasis on controlled movements and minimal impact, Wall Pilates is kinder to the joints and suitable for a larger age range.

3. Perfect Posture: Bad posture might eventually cause discomfort and agony. With a focus on spinal alignment, Wall Pilates helps women over 40 correct and maintain healthy posture, lowering their chance of developing chronic back pain.

4. Core Strength: The cornerstone of Pilates, and Wall Pilates is no exception, is core strength. A strong core is essential for daily tasks and can help prevent lower back pain, which is a typical worry as we get older.

5. Mind-Body Connection: Pilates is a mind-body discipline, not just a physical one. Pilates on the wall promotes awareness by emphasizing breath management and mental attention. Positive effects on stress reduction and mental clarity may result from this.

6. Wall Pilates is adaptable to different fitness levels, making it appropriate for both beginning and advanced practitioners. With this flexibility, women over 40 can develop at their own rate and customize the practice to meet their own needs.

7. Social Connection: Group Wall Pilates lessons give women over 40 the chance to meet people who have similar fitness aspirations. In terms of inspiration and companionship, a sense of belonging and support can be important.

In conclusion, Pilates, in all of its varieties, has a wealth of advantages for women over 40. Wall Pilates distinguishes out as a fantastic option with its distinctive blend of support, moderate exercises, and attention on posture. It's more than simply a workout; it's a route to renewal, empowerment, and overall wellbeing. Consider the transforming potential of Wall Pilates as you begin your fitness journey or look to improve your current regimen. Wall Pilates is the haven where power, elegance, and vitality converge.

Day 1:

Exercise: Wall Sit

Instructions: Stand with your back against the wall and lower into a seated position, with knees at a 90-degree angle. Hold for 40 seconds and repeat 4 times.

Day 2:

Exercise: Wall Roll-Down

Instructions: Stand tall with your back against the wall, slowly roll down to touch your toes, and then roll back up. Repeat 8-10 times.

Day 3:

Exercise: Wall Plank

Instructions: Assume a plank position with your forearms against the wall, body straight. Hold for thirty five seconds and then repeat four times.

Day 4:

Exercise: Wall Bridge

Instructions: Lie on your back with feet on the wall, lift your hips off the ground, and hold for 20 seconds. Lower down and repeat 5 times.

Day 5:

Exercise: Wall Push-Ups

Instructions: Stand facing the wall, place your hands shoulder-width apart, and perform push-ups against the wall. Do 10-12 reps.

Day 6:

Exercise: Wall Squats with Ball Squeeze

Instructions: Place a small ball between your knees and perform wall squats, squeezing the ball. Do 12-15 squats.

Day 7:

Rest Day

Day 8:

Exercise: Wall Teaser

Instructions: Lie on your back with legs against the wall, reach your arms overhead, and perform a teaser motion. Do 8-10 reps.

Day 9:

Exercise: Wall Side Leg Lifts

Instructions: Stand sideways to the wall, lift your top leg to the side, and lower it back down. Repeat 12-15 times per leg.

Day 10:

Exercise: Wall Spine Stretch

Instructions: Sit close to the wall with legs extended, reach forward to touch your toes, and roll back up. Repeat 8-10 times.

Day 11:

Exercise: Wall Ball Pike

Instructions: Assume a plank position with feet on a ball against the wall, pike your hips upward. Do 8-10 repetitions.

Day 12:

Rest Day

Day 13:

Exercise: Wall Calf Raises

Instructions: Stand facing the wall, lift onto your toes, and lower down. Repeat 15-20 times.

Day 14:

Exercise: Wall Backbend

Instructions: Stand with your back to the wall, arch backward, and place your hands on the wall. Endure for twenty one seconds, then gently repeat four times.

Day 15:

Exercise: Wall Leg Press

Instructions: Lie on your back, place your feet against the wall, and press your legs straight. Do 10-12 repetitions.

Day 16:

Exercise: Wall Oblique Twist

Instructions: Sit on the floor, lean back against the wall, and twist your torso side to side. Repeat 12-15 times per side.

Day 17:

Rest Day

Day 18:

Exercise: Wall Scissor

Instructions: Lie on your back with legs against the wall, crisscross your legs in a scissor motion. Repeat 10-12 times.

Day 19:

Exercise: Wall Single Leg Circle

Instructions: Lie on your back, extend one leg toward the ceiling, and make circles with your foot. Do 8-10 circles per leg.

Day 20:

Exercise: Wall Roll-Up

Instructions: Sit on the floor, press your back against the wall, and roll up to touch your toes. Roll back down and repeat 8-10 times.

Day 21:

Exercise: Wall V-Sit

Instructions: Sit on the floor with your back against the wall, lift your legs and torso into a V position. Endure for twenty one seconds then repeat four times.

Day 22:

Rest Day

Day 23:

Exercise: Wall Toe Taps

Instructions: Lie on your back with feet against the wall, tap one foot on the wall at a time. Repeat 15-20 times per leg.

Day 24:

Exercise: Wall Lunge

Instructions: Stand with one foot against the wall, perform lunges by bending your knee. Do 10-12 lunges per leg.

Day 25:

Exercise: Wall Tabletop
Instructions: Sit on the floor, press your hands against the wall, and lift your hips off the ground. Hold for twenty one seconds, then repeat 4 times.

Circles of Wall Arms:

Standing with your arms out to the sides, face the wall.
Use your arms to move in little circles.
12–15 rounds in both directions should be repeated.

Resistance band leg lifts against the wall:

At ankle height, fasten a resistance band to the wall.
Standing perpendicular to the wall, wrap the other end over your ankle and secure.
As you lift your leg away from the resistance band, extend it.
On each leg, repeat 12 to 15 times.

The wall tricep dip:

Knees bent, lean back against the wall while you sit on the floor.

With your fingers pointed in the direction of the wall, place your hands on the ground behind you.

To lower your body, raise your hips off the floor and flex your elbows.

Repeat 10–12 times, then push yourself back up.

Cat-Cow Stretch on a Wall:

Put your hands on the wall at shoulder height while standing with your back to the wall.

Take a breath as you assume the "Cow" position, arching your back away from the wall.

As you assume the cat stance, exhale as you turn your back toward the wall.

Eight to ten times, repeat this stretch.

Knee tucks while doing a wall plank:

Assume a plank position with your body straight and forearms up against the wall.
One at a time, alternately bring each knee to your chest.
On each leg, perform 12 to 15 knee tucks.

Passing a wall ball:

Holding a little ball in your hands, sit on the floor with your back to the wall.
Pass the ball from your hands to your feet while standing up straight.
Repeat the motion for 10 to 12 times before passing it again.

Quadruped Leg Lifts on a Wall:

Kneel with your hands on the wall and your back to the wall.
Lift one leg behind you and maintain a 90-degree bend in it.
On each leg, repeat for 12 to 15 lifts.

Aside the wall:

With your feet up against the wall and your elbow
just under your shoulder, lie on your side.
form a straight line from your heels up to your head
by elavating/lifting your hips off the floor.
Hold the position for 20 seconds on each side, then
switch.

Russian twist on a wall

Kneel on the floor with your back against the wall
and your feet just off the floor.
With both hands holding a little ball, turn your body
to contact the ball to the wall on either side.
Twist 12 to 15 times on each side.

Wall Stretch in Child's Pose:

Kneel with your back to the wall and your palms on
the surface.
Stretching your arms and torso against the wall,
lean back onto your heels.
If necessary, continue this soothing stretch for 30
seconds.

Congratulations on completing the 30-day wall Pilates challenge! Remember to listen to your body, take breaks as needed, and consult a fitness professional if you have any concerns or injuries. Happy exercising!

4-WEEKS EXERCISE PLAN

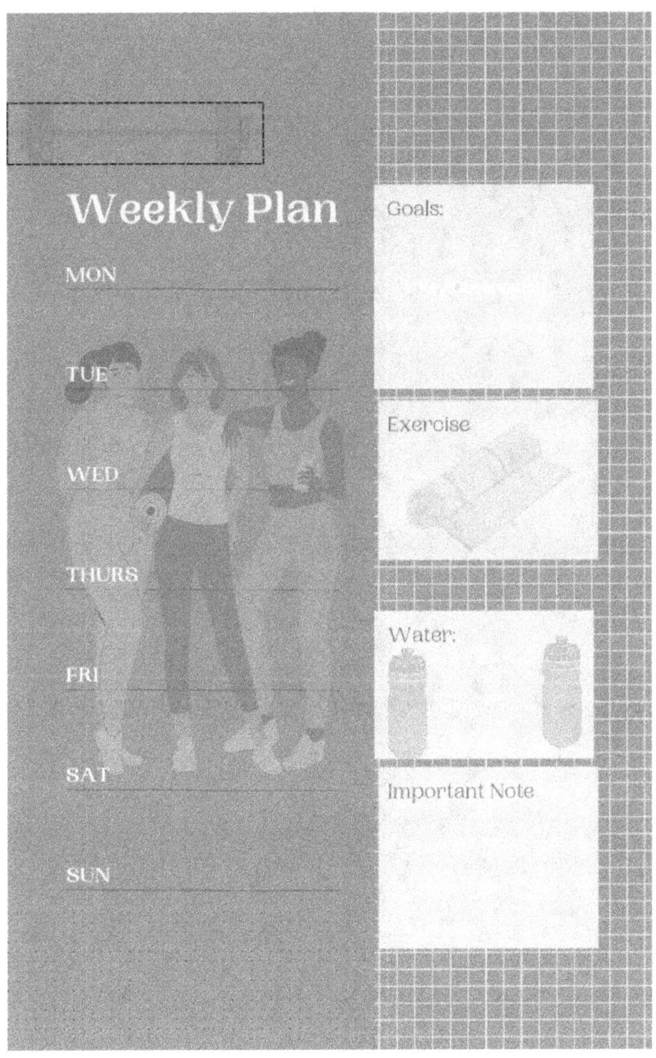

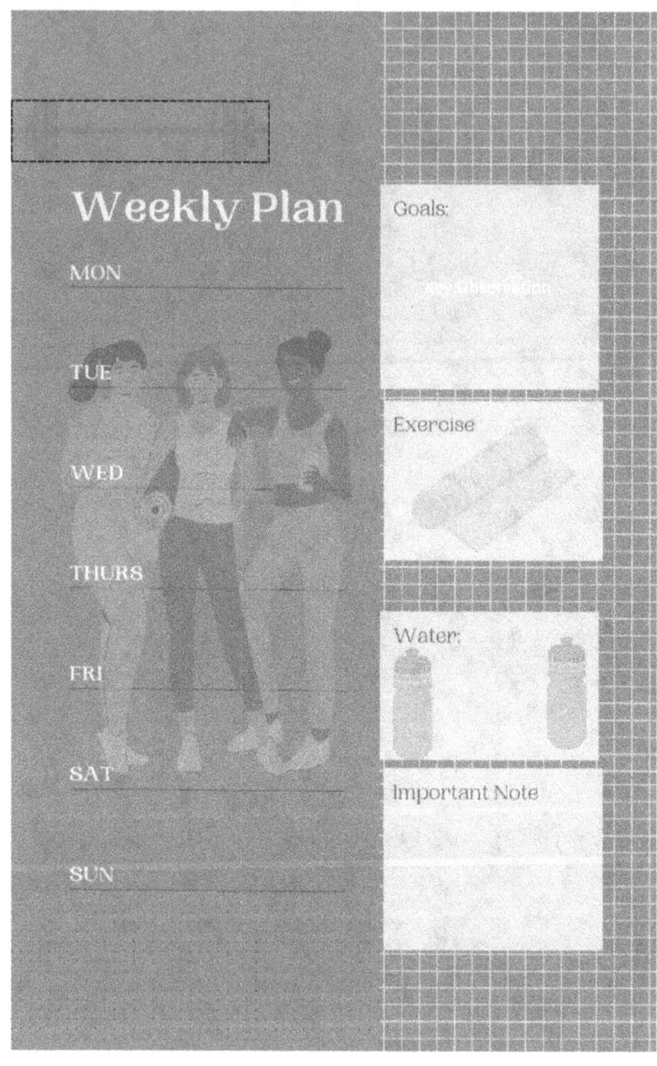
Weekly Plan
MON
TUE
WED
THURS
FRI
SAT
SUN
Goals:
Exercise
Water:
Important Note

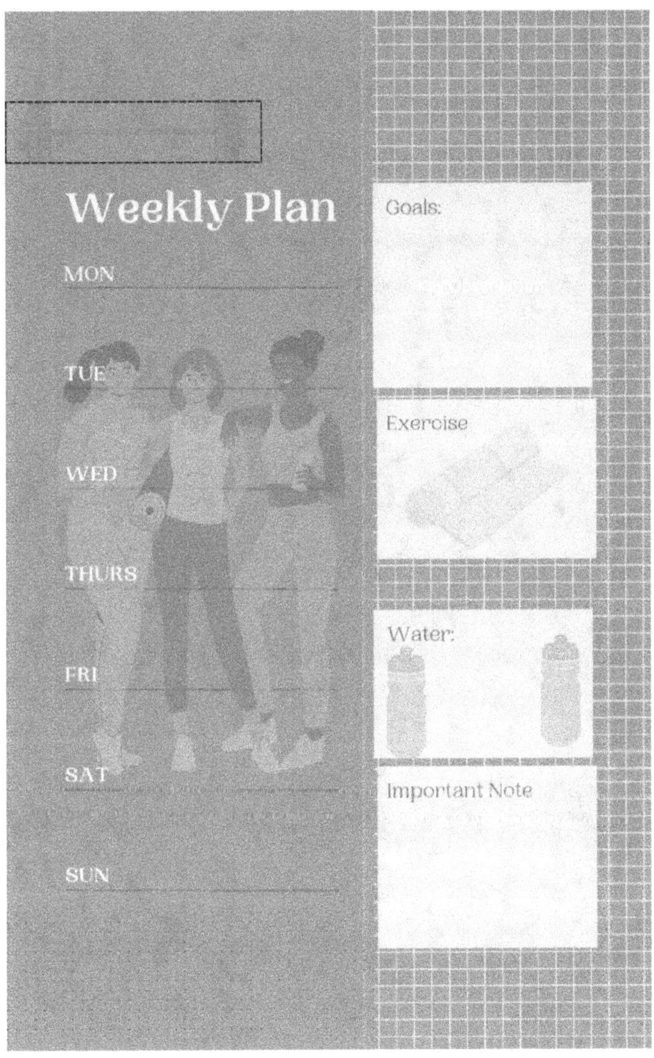
Weekly Plan
MON
TUE
WED
THURS
FRI
SAT
SUN
Goals:
Exercise
Water:
Important Note

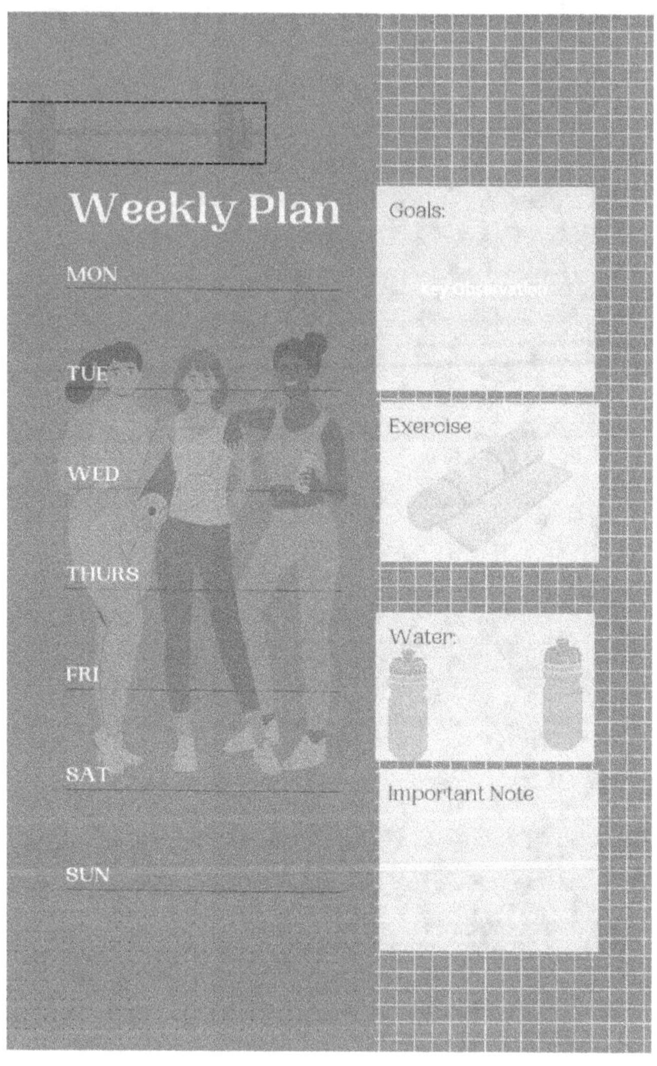
Weekly Plan
MON
TUE
WED
THURS
FRI
SAT
SUN
Goals:
Key Observation
Exercise
Water:
Important Note

Exercise Daily Log

28

EXERCISE LOG

MONTH OF :

DATE	PRE-EXERCISE MEAL/SNACK	ENERGY LEVEL BEFORE	ACTIVITY/EXERCISE	TIME

www.ingramcontent.com/pod-product-compliance
Lightning Source LLC
Chambersburg PA
CBHW070756260726
48660CB00007B/3155